AROMATHERAPY
FOR HORSES

by
Caroline Ingraham EAA

Foreword by
Tim Couzens BVetMed, MRCVS, VetMFHom

Illustrations by
Carole Vincer

KENILWORTH PRESS

First published in Great Britain by
The Kenilworth Press Limited,
Addington, Buckingham, MK18 2JR

British Library Cataloguing in Publication Data
A catalogue record for this book is available from the British Library.

ISBN 1-872082-98-X

Typeset by The Kenilworth Press Limited

Printed in Great Britain by Westway Offset, Wembley

Important note
Veterinary Surgeons Act, 1966; Medicines Act, 1968; Cruelty to Animals Act, 1911

Only a qualified veterinary surgeon may legally treat or prescribe for your horse. If an owner consults a non-vet and thereby fails to alleviate suffering for his or her animal, prosecution under the 1911 act is a possibility.

This book is not intended as a substitute for the medical advice of veterinarians. The reader should consult a veterinary surgeon regularly in matters relating to his or her horse's health, and particularly in respect of any symptoms which may require diagnosis or medical attention. No responsibility can be taken by the author, publishers or distributors of this book for the application of any of the enclosed information in practice.

CONTENTS

Foreword

by Tim Couzens BVetMed, MRCVS, VetMFHom

There are a great many books about aromatherapy, but what makes this work so unique and fascinating is the way in which essential oils can be used to treat horses, adding another perspective to the growing popularity of complementary equine therapies.

It is not suprising to find that horses respond so well to aromatherapy. This delicate and fragrant healing art taps directly into the refined and fine-tuned energy of these sensitive animals, reflecting the very qualities of the oils themselves.

This book not only reveals the subtle, gentle and often miraculous ways in which aromatherapy can work, but also explains the properties and characteristics of individual oils.

Using this basic knowledge and working with your horse's own instincts, you can treat a wide range of common conditions both safely and effectively with this powerful form of natural therapy.

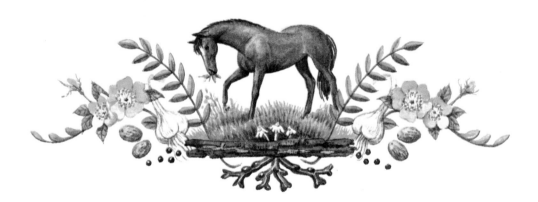

How to use this book

1. Read the whole book thoroughly at least once before starting.
2. Turn to page 8 – 'Selecting oils for a particular condition'.
3. Refer to pages 22-23 – 'Quick-reference selection charts'.
4. Turn to page 9 to assess the horse's response.
5. Read up on the oils that are needed – pages 20-21.
6. Blend the oils as on page 10 – 'Doses and dilutions'.
7. Follow the guidelines on applications and reactions on pages 12-14.
8. **Always follow the recommendations on safety given on page 11.**

Ancient art – new science

What is aromatherapy?

Aromatherapy is the use of essential oils to improve physical and emotional well-being.

Essential oils are concentrated medicines extracted mainly by distillation from herbs, flowers, gums, fruits, roots and seeds. They possess individual qualities that can heal and balance various ailments within the mind and body.

Essential oils can work very quickly. Their effects are often noticed within days of treatment and sometimes immediately after application.

When a horse is unwell, suffering from a physical or emotional disorder, it will, in its natural habitat, seek out the correct plant or herb to restore its health. Today, however, most horses do not have this freedom of choice and need to rely on us for their well-being.

Aromatherapy offers a form of treatment that allows the horse and its carer to combine their efforts in the healing process as the horse actively participates in the selection of the oils that are needed.

Ancient to modern

The Ancient Egyptian priests were among the first to gain an in-depth understanding of aromatics. They dispensed them for their medicinal properties by matching the plant's shape and colour to the condition occurring in the body. For example, plants with purple flowering tops such as Lavender were used for their sedative properties, and red plants such as Cinnamon were used for their stimulating properties. Leaves, regarded as the lungs of the earth, were used to treat respiratory disorders, whilst roots were used for grounding and sedating.

In the nineteenth century it was discovered that micro-organisms were the cause of many diseases. It was also noticed that there was a low incidence of tuberculosis in the flower-growing districts in France, which led to the first laboratory tests on the antibacterial properties of essential oils. In 1887, studies from France showed that the micro-organisms of glandular fever and yellow fever were easily killed when exposed to a selection of anti-bacterial and anti-viral oils, and so essential oils soon became an important part of every veterinary surgeon's and doctor's bag.

It was the prominent French chemist, René-Maurice Gattefossé, who actually coined the name 'aromatherapy' due to the ability of certain oils to disinfect the air. He did much research on essential oils, noting that some of them had a greater antiseptic value than many oils that had been synthetically reconstructed.

One of his discoveries was that a burn treated with Lavender oil healed surprisingly quickly, leaving no infection or scar. He also wrote a book on essential oils in 1937.

The use of essential oils declined in the middle of the twentieth century due to the production of synthetic drugs, many of which were actually based on the molecular structure of essential oils. These new drugs appeared to act more effectively and offered guaranteed availability and cost, but being constructed of synthetic materials they do not contain the important life-force that is found within nature.

However, science is now taking a fresh look at these natural oils, identifying their powerful healing properties.

What are essential oils?

Essential oils are found in tiny sacs on the surface of plant tissue. Most are extracted by distillation, but some, like citrus fruits for example, are cold pressed. Distillation can considerably change the chemical make-up of the original plant oil, producing a very concentrated and powerful remedy.

The oils affect bodily functions in various ways depending on which oils are chosen and how they are used. Applied to the skin they are one of the few substances that will pass through the dermal layers and into the bloodstream. They also have the ability to evaporate into the air allowing the aroma to reach the emotional centre of the brain. The nose can smell and identify thousands of different chemical compounds. These are thought to be transferred into messages that are sent to various parts of the brain where mood and bodily function may be affected.

Each essential oil has a specific response to various disorders. Using the correct oil a variety of conditions can often be successfully helped. Allergies, skin disorders, laminitis, arthritis, aches and sprains, immune disorders, respiratory problems and emotional disorders, are some of the many problems treated with essential oils. **It must be stressed, however, that veterinary advice must first be sought**.

Essential oils offer a life energy that works like a catalyst, allowing the oil to discriminate which areas need balancing, stimulating, sedating or healing. For example: Rose oil can help bring mares into season yet can also calm mares that are overly marish. Thus they can act as a natural balancing agent.

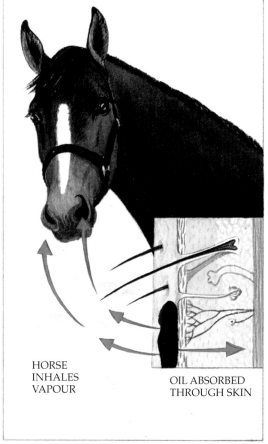

HORSE INHALES VAPOUR

OIL ABSORBED THROUGH SKIN

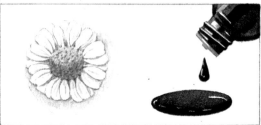

Many of the constituents present in the oils are not found in the plant's original form. German Chamomile and Yarrow plants, for example, are not blue in colour, yet during distillation they produce dark blue azulene. The azulene gives the oils their strong antiseptic and anti-inflammatory properties.

The horse's sense of smell

Horses are very sensitive to smell. It is important in the selection of food and medicine, in the detection of predators, to bond mother and foal, to influence sexual behaviour and aids in recognising locations.

Horses instinctively smell essential oils in the correct way. They will first smell with one nostril, which connects to one side of the brain, and then will turn (if the oil interests them) and smell with the other nostril, which connects to the other side of the brain. If the aroma offers no therapeutic value the horse will turn away from it.

Horses will often show more interest in the therapist's selection of oils than in their feed or carrots.

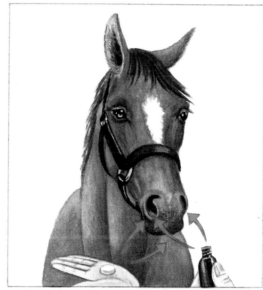

Some horses with a passion for mints will show a preference for Peppermint essential oil, as opposed to mints, when both are offered at the same time.

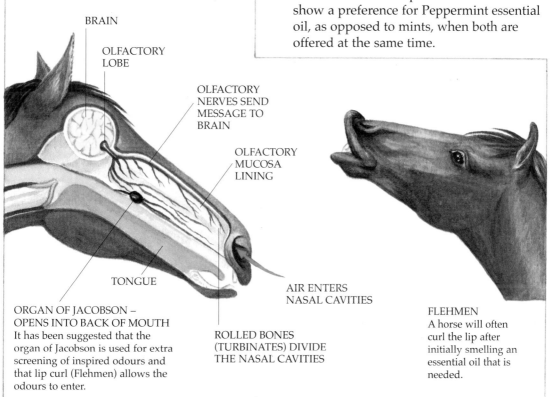

BRAIN

OLFACTORY LOBE

OLFACTORY NERVES SEND MESSAGE TO BRAIN

OLFACTORY MUCOSA LINING

TONGUE

AIR ENTERS NASAL CAVITIES

ORGAN OF JACOBSON – OPENS INTO BACK OF MOUTH
It has been suggested that the organ of Jacobson is used for extra screening of inspired odours and that lip curl (Flehmen) allows the odours to enter.

ROLLED BONES (TURBINATES) DIVIDE THE NASAL CAVITIES

FLEHMEN
A horse will often curl the lip after initially smelling an essential oil that is needed.

Selecting oils for a particular condition

Example 1

DATE 26·5·97   NAME *Freya*.

AGE *11 years*.   BREED *Thoroughbred*.

MAIN COMPLAINT
Very tense. Spooks easily out riding.

PAST ILLNESS RECURRING PROBLEMS
Mud Fever. Stress-related colic. Itchy, flaky skin.

TEMPERAMENT and OTHER INFORMATION
Good-natured horse. Nervous. Owned her for six years; not much known about her past.

FEED *Oats. Chaff. Flaked barley. Sugar beet pulp.*

STABLING *In at night.*

HOOF CONDITION *Good.*

Example 2

DATE *9·8·97*   NAME *Harris*.

AGE *8 years*.   BREED *Welsh Cob*.

MAIN COMPLAINT
C.O.P.D. Run Down.

PAST ILLNESS RECURRING PROBLEMS
Laminitis.

TEMPERAMENT and OTHER PROBLEMS
Lethargic. Owned him for four years. Before then had changed hands many times. Had been neglected as a yearling.

FEED *Chaff. Nuts.*

STABLING *Out in Summer. In at night in Winter.*

HOOF CONDITION *Poor.*

Here are two examples illlustrating general guidelines for the selection of oils. In addition to the complaint, the horse's temperament should always be assessed and appropriate oils offered. If the horse shows little interest in the oils chosen, look through the lists and try another selection.

Example 1

1. Assess main complaint: recurring colic; skin; nervousness.
2. Refer to charts on pages 22-23: skin and stomach problems of a nervous origin = Roman Chamomile.
3. Not much known about horse's past. There may be suppressed trauma = Rose. (If available perhaps also try Yarrow to help with the release.)
4. Tense / spooks easily: try Violet Leaf, Jasmine, Frankincense or Clary Sage. If, however, the horse responds to Roman Chamomile, it will probably cover all the above symptoms.

Example 2

1. Assess complaint: COPD; run down; lethargic.
2. Refer to charts on pages 22-23: respiratory, immune stimulants, general stimulants, anti-inflammatory oils, behavioural / emotional oils.
3. Lungs and lethargy = Peppermint – very stimulating to central nervous system and lungs; opens up airways. A good first choice.
4. Conditions involving a possible histamine reaction, such as in COPD and laminitis = Great Mugwort.
5. Run down; poor hoof condition = Carrot Seed; Seaweed; Garlic.
6. Neglected = Rose or Neroli. Change of home / stable yard = Violet Leaf.

Testing the response

1. Offer each aroma that you have selected for the horse – not more than five aromas at one time. Wait approx. 20 minutes before offering others.

2. Make a note of the response.

- Smells with interest/flares both nostrils. *Offer the oils twice daily before possible application.*

- Tries to nibble at the bottle. (Make sure that the bottle is held firmly so that the horse cannot snatch it out of your hand.) *Offer the oils twice daily before possible application.*

- Curls lips (flehmen). *Offer the oils twice daily before possible application.*

- Smells with just one nostril. (Each nostril connects to the opposite side of the brain. In this case, the blend could be massaged around that particular nostril). *Offer the oils once daily before possible application.*

- Shows only slight interest, then turns away. This could indicate that the aroma itself is all that is needed to trigger a reaction, or that your horse may be suited to other oils. *Offer once daily before possible application.*

- Turns head away/ears back. *Do not apply.*

The cause of the problem must always be addressed. The oils can usually help release past issues and balance emotional states etc. but if the problem is on-going, such as an ill-fitting saddle or a stable without a view, the oils may help but they will not make the problem go away.

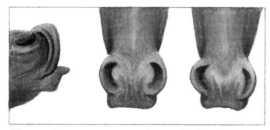

Choose between one to five oils that have received the greatest interest.

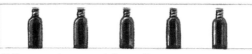

Offer maximum of five oils at any one time.

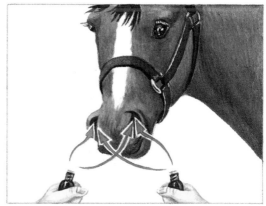

If unsure of the preference of any two oils, allow the horse to smell the aroma of each, then hold the bottles approximately one to two feet apart. The horse will turn to the oil for which he has the greater need. If both oils are going to be used in the blend, allow the preferred aroma to be slightly stronger.

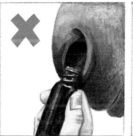 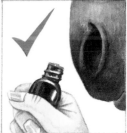

Do **not** touch nose with bottle.

Doses and dilutions

The practice of aromatherapy is a matter of understanding the oils and the individual treatment. The amounts suggested are, therefore, guidelines. Each horse's needs will vary depending on the degree and nature of the problem. Old, young, chronically ill and sensitive horses will need blends that are diluted further than recommended here.

Base oils/carrier oils

Base (carrier) oils do not contain any essential oils. **Grapeseed** is a light oil, less oily than most other base oils. **Walnut** and **apricot kernel** have a high absorption rate. **Jojoba** is useful for mixing into essential oils that are to be pre-blended due to its non-oxidising properties.

Other suitable oils: avocado, hazelnut, kukui, passion flower, peach kernel and sweet almond.

The aim of blending is to select the correct oil or combination of oils that will suit the individual horse. Some essential oils are stronger than others, which is apparent from their aroma. Try not to blend more than three oils in one blend. Blend the oils so that the ones that have achieved the greatest interest have a stronger aroma. Try to keep floral oils in one blend, antiseptic oils in another, and food oils in another. If in doubt, blend each oil separately. Apply the stimulating oils, such as Peppermint, in the morning, and sedative ones in the evening. If, however, the horse needs calming during the day then use the sedatives.

Formulas given in the back of the book are for a specific use, therefore stronger.

1ml = 20 drops	5ml = 100 drops (1 teaspoon)
	15ml = 1 tablespoon

APPLICATION TO NOSTRILS: DILUTE IN A BASE OIL

Approximately 5-7 drops of essential oil in 12ml base oil. If using more than one essential oil, the total number of drops should still add up to approximately the same amount.

APPLICATION TO COAT, WOUNDS AND IRRITATED SKIN IN A WATER-BASED GEL

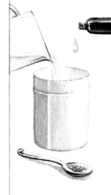

To 2 teaspoons of gel add approx. 30ml of water. If it separates, continued whisking should bind it together. For use on a larger area add 60-90ml water.

Add approximately 10-15 drops of essential oil to 50ml of gel. If using more than one essential oil the total number of drops should still be approx. 10-15.

APPLICATION TO FOOD: DILUTE IN A BASE OIL

Add one drop of essential oil to 1ml of base oil or 5% dilution.

Add approximately 5-6 drops of blended essential oil to carrot or add to a handful of feed, or allow to lick off hand.

For Garlic and Thyme, add no more than 3-4 drops to 10ml of base oil.

SHAMPOO AND COMPRESS

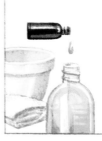

Add 10-15 drops of essential oil to 50ml shampoo or warm water. Shake or agitate well. When applying to sensitive skins or when using Garlic or Thyme, use half the amount of essential oil – 5-7 drops to 50ml of water (4-5 drops of Yarrow or German Chamomile will help to counteract the harsh effects of Garlic on the skin).

Safety

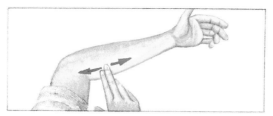

Patch-test all blends before their application by dabbing a small amount onto the inside of the elbow. If itching or redness occurs dilute further.

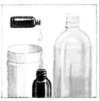
Dilute all essential oils in base oil, plain gel, aloe vera gel, shampoo or warm water, except those listed below for wounds.

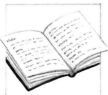
Read up on each oil before application.

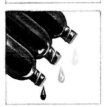
Oils which can be used undiluted on simple wounds are: Lavender, Tea Tree, Yarrow and German Chamomile.

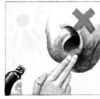
Do not apply to the nostrils, in an oil base in direct sunlight. It may cause sunburn.

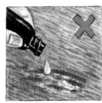
Do not use base oil on wounds, irritated skin, mud fever or sweet itch.

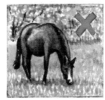
Caution: Do not use essential oils on in-foal mares unless directed by your vet.

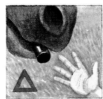
Caution: Hold the bottle firmly. The horse may try to snatch it out of your hand with his mouth.

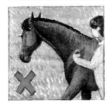
If the horse rejects an oil don't force it upon him. Before each application test the horse's response to the aroma.

1. Veterinary approval needs to be sought before essential oil application.
2. Do not allow bottles of undiluted essential oil to touch the nostrils.
3. Treat all essential oils with the same respect as over-the-counter medications.
4. High doses of essential oils (10-20mls) taken internally could result in poisoning.
5. Stop if adverse reactions appear. Refer to page 14.
6. Do not apply for longer than 2 weeks without further professional advice.
7. Do not use essential oils around the eyes or genital area.
8. It is very important to work 'with' the horse – never force him to accept an oil he rejects. Applying oils that are not wanted could actually bring on the symptoms that they would normally alleviate.
9. Do not balance essential oil bottles on stable doors or places where they may easily fall and break.

Applications

External application

If the horse is very keen on the aroma, apply selected oil twice daily to the **nostrils** and/or **poll area,** or allow him to **lick it off your hand.** Other areas of the body may also benefit from direct application, depending on the condition (see illustrations). The horse will show you his dislikes by turning away or putting his ears back as you make the application. However, all areas may be enjoyed equally. Remember: test the horse's response to the aroma before each application.

When the interest is moderate apply once daily until the horse turns away from the aroma. At this stage the condition should have improved or cleared. If the condition has not completely cleared, it may be that an underlying issue still needs to be treated.

Discontinue treatment if no improvement is seen within the first two weeks, regardless of the interest the horse has to the oil. Seek professional advice.

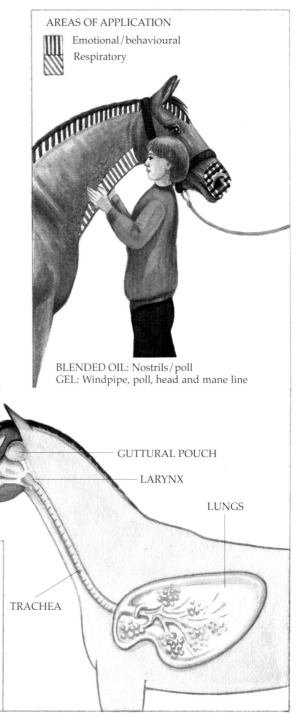

AREAS OF APPLICATION

▦ Emotional/behavioural

▨ Respiratory

BLENDED OIL: Nostrils/poll
GEL: Windpipe, poll, head and mane line

RESPIRATORY TRACT

SINUSES

GUTTURAL POUCH

NASAL CHAMBERS

LARYNX

LUNGS

TRACHEA

INHALATION USING A NOSE BAG

Put a layer of hay in a nose bag. Add a total of 10-15 drops of essential oil to half a litre (1 pint) of hot or boiling water and pour over hay. Cover with more hay so that nose of the horse will not burn or be uncomfortably hot.

Oral application

The food oils such as Carrot Seed, Garlic and Seaweed are usually associated with the treatment of conditions within the body and have a similar pH to that of the horse's gut. **They should, however, only be given under veterinary advice.**

If the horse is very keen on the aroma offer it twice daily until the interest lessens, then offer it once daily until there is no further interest in the oil.

Do not apply for more than two weeks without seeking further professional advice. If no improvement is seen within this time, stop the application.

Topical application

Use on isolated areas for conditions such as: sweet itch, mud fever, arthritis, aches and sprains, and wounds

Do **not** use base oils on wounds or irritated skin. Use a compress, water-based gel or aloe vera gel. (Use the aloe vera gel in the same way as the water-based gel; however, dilution with water is optional.) Tea Tree, Lavender, German Chamomile or Yarrow may be used undiluted on wounds in certain cases (see page 17).

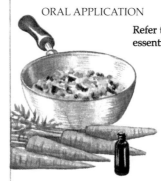

ORAL APPLICATION

Refer to charts for suitable essential oils.

Approximately 6 drops of blended essential oil on a carrot or in feed, once or twice daily, for a maximum of 2 weeks.

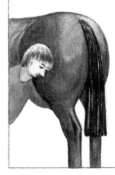

APPLICATION AREAS FOR BLADDER AND STOMACH PROBLEMS

Apply oils on belly area in between legs (where the skin is exposed).
Apply in an oil base 1-2 times daily, maximum 2 weeks. Caution: avoid genital area.

If the horse does not like to be touched in an area, do not apply oil there. Offer another form of application instead.

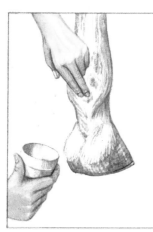

TOPICAL APPLICATION

In the case of SWEET ITCH AND MUD FEVER, apply gel two times daily for 3-5 days then once daily or as needed.

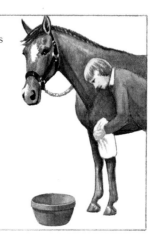

COMPRESS – useful for topical applications

Add a total of 6-10 drops of essential oil to a bowl of approximately $^1/_4$ - $^1/_2$ pint of luke warm water. Agitate well, immerse cloth, wring out excess water and apply to the area.

Reactions

Positive reactions from essential oils can normally be seen within the first three to seven days of treatment but can also occur immediately after their application. The length of time varies depending on the nature of the illness and the individual horse. The effects may be more immediate when treating acute conditions than when dealing with chronic (long-standing) ones. In most cases the oils will stimulate the body's own healing process.

Sometimes, however, a healing crisis may occur causing the symptoms to worsen. This is a cleansing process that may occur in the first few days of treatment and should last no longer than two or three days. Should symptoms appear to worsen for longer than this, stop application and seek professional help.

Each horse will have an individual response and preference for the application of the oils. Some may choose only external application, whereas others may prefer to lick the blend off the hand and back away from physical application; many will choose and enjoy all forms of application. Be aware that his preferences may change. The horse guides the treatment as to which oils are needed, their application and how often.

It is very important to work 'with' the horse. If the horse does not appear very interested in any essential oils it may be that the wrong oils have been chosen or that he or his problem is not suited to aromatherapy and may benefit from another form of treatment such as homoeopathy or herbal medicine.

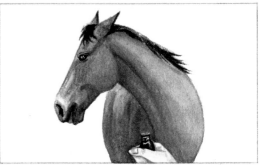

Turning away or ears back indicates that the horse does not want application to a particular area.

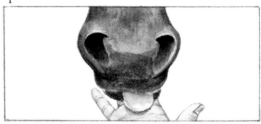

Some horses prefer to lick the oil off the hand using the back of the tongue.

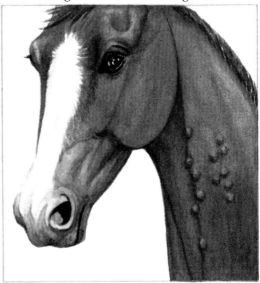

Lumps on the neck might indicate an allergic reaction. Should this happen stop all essential oil application. If they do not disappear within a couple of days, call vet.

Behavioural problems

This is a guide to the oils that may be needed for common problems.

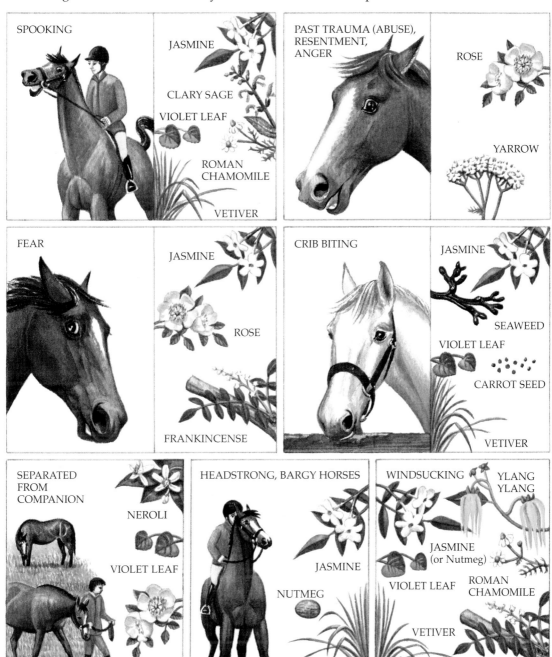

SPOOKING

JASMINE

CLARY SAGE

VIOLET LEAF

ROMAN CHAMOMILE

VETIVER

PAST TRAUMA (ABUSE), RESENTMENT, ANGER

ROSE

YARROW

FEAR

JASMINE

ROSE

FRANKINCENSE

CRIB BITING

JASMINE

SEAWEED

VIOLET LEAF

CARROT SEED

VETIVER

SEPARATED FROM COMPANION

NEROLI

VIOLET LEAF

ROSE

HEADSTRONG, BARGY HORSES

JASMINE

NUTMEG

VETIVER

WINDSUCKING

YLANG YLANG

JASMINE (or Nutmeg)

VIOLET LEAF

ROMAN CHAMOMILE

VETIVER

FRANKINCENSE

First aid

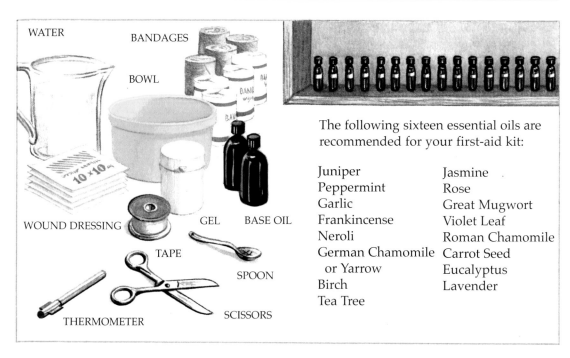

WATER
BANDAGES
BOWL
WOUND DRESSING
GEL   BASE OIL
TAPE
SPOON
THERMOMETER
SCISSORS

The following sixteen essential oils are recommended for your first-aid kit:

Juniper	Jasmine
Peppermint	Rose
Garlic	Great Mugwort
Frankincense	Violet Leaf
Neroli	Roman Chamomile
German Chamomile	Carrot Seed
or Yarrow	Eucalyptus
Birch	Lavender
Tea Tree	

FIRST AID FOR ACHES AND SPRAINS (also useful for arthritis)

	DROPS	ACTION
Peppermint	30	Deep heat. Ice-pack effect. Anti-inflammatory.
Birch	10	Helps break down lactic acid (waste product of muscles that can cause stiffness and pain).
Juniper	10	Helps clear the system of toxins and excess water retention. Effective for arthritis.
Yarrow	4	Anti-inflammatory to swollen tissues.

Blend into 100ml of gel or base oil.

Patch test should offer feeling of hot and cold. Slightly numbing.	✖ Do not apply to broken skin.

Wounds

The oils recommended here are suitable for wounds that do not require veterinary attention - if in doubt consult your vet. Veterinary advice should always be sought if a wound is over one inch long because it may need stitches.

Do **not** apply any of these oils in a base oil as it will not allow the wound to dry.

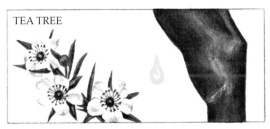

Tea Tree is a natural antibiotic and contains four constituents not found anywhere else in nature. It is highly antiseptic, antifungal and antiviral. It is very effective in the cleansing of wounds. An Australian study reported that 'Tea Tree essential oil is thirteen times stronger than carbolic acid', which was once used as a major antiseptic. It also stated that 'Tea Tree is a non-poisonous, non irritant antiseptic of unusual strength'.

Another study reports that 'applying Tea Tree oil to pus-filled infections, dissolved the pus and left the surface of the infected wounds clean without any apparent irritation to healthy tissues'. It was also noted that in the presence of blood, pus and other foreign matter, the antiseptic properties of the oil were increased by 10-12%.

Apply undiluted Tea Tree to the wound, or use it in a plain or aloe vera gel, or in a compress soaked in a Tea Tree solution. The wound needs to be dressed twice daily, then, as signs of healing begin, once daily until it is dry to the touch and has no signs of oozing. At this stage apply Lavender.

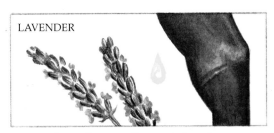

Lavender offers antibacterial and analgesic properties but it is more renowned for its ability to accelerate the regeneration of healthy skin cells, minimising scarring.

Apply undiluted to the area or use in a water-based or aloe vera gel, or via a compress.

Lavender will also deter flies.

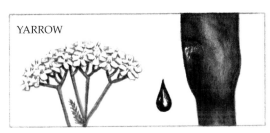

Yarrow. Azulene, the constituent responsible for the blue colour in this essential oil, contains powerful anti-inflammatory and antibacterial properties while also having a soothing action on skin tissues, neutralising excess heat and pain. It also acts like a protective dressing and is a very effective stimulant to the healing process.

Apply undiluted on the wound. Do not dilute in a base material. This oil is more effective in its undiluted state for this type of condition.

German Chamomile may be used as an alternative to Yarrow.

Skin problems

FLY REPELLENT FORMULA

Lavender	20 drops
Tea tree	20 drops
Eucalyptus	20 drops
Garlic	7 drops

Shake well and store in a glass bottle.

Spray: Add 60 drops (3ml) of the blend to 200ml water in a spray bottle.(A disperser – supplied by essential oil specialists – can help to infuse the oil and water.)

Wipe: Add 30-40 drops to half litre (1 pint) of warm water. Mix well. Apply using a sponge or cloth, squeeze out excess water, wipe over coat in direction of the hair. Use once or twice daily. Avoid contact with the eyes.

INSECT BITES

Apply 1-2 drops of undiluted Yarrow, German Chamomile or Tea Tree oil to the bite, twice daily. For sensitive skins mix the oil with aloe vera gel.

SWEET ITCH FORMULA

Lavender	10 drops
Tea Tree	10 drops
Roman Chamomile	5 drops
Yarrow/German Chamomile	5 drops
Garlic	5 drops (or 3-4 capsules)

Add formula to 100ml of plain or aloe vera gel (do not blend in a base oil). Apply once or twice daily, for a maximum of 2-3 weeks. Seek professional advice for continued use.

MUD FEVER FORMULA

Lavender	10 drops
Tea Tree	20 drops
Roman Chamomile	5 drops
Yarrow/German Chamomile	5 drops
Garlic	4 drops

Add formula to 100ml of plain or aloe vera gel (do not blend in a base oil). Apply once or twice daily, for maximum 2-3 weeks. Seek professional advice for continued use.

THRUSH

Ensure that the horse is kept in a clean, dry area. Ask your farrier to trim the horse's frogs and remove dead tissue. Apply undiluted Tea Tree twice daily until condition clears.

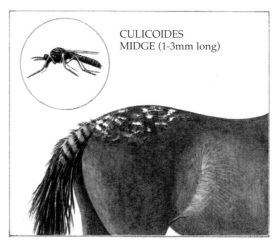

CULICOIDES MIDGE (1-3mm long)

Sweet itch is an allergic reaction to Culicoides midges. It causes severe skin irritation resulting in itching and raw, bald patches.

Travelling

Travelling often causes the horse to brace itself in very unnatural positions for long periods of time. The constant strain on the muscles causes them to release lactic acid, a waste product that can cause stiffness, pain and even muscle damage.

If the muscles are stiff the horse's performance is likely to suffer. The areas usually involved are the shoulders, back, quarters and upper legs. These can be washed down using the travel wash blend given below.

Problems with loading

Loading difficulties are common and can be very distressing to all involved. Refer to the section on behavioural/emotional oils, page 22, for appropriate selection. Make a blend of the oil or oils that when offered have received the most interest. Add them to a base oil and apply to the nostrils and/or poll area. Start the treatment a week before the horse is to be boxed. Continue applying the oils until there is no longer an interest in them. If the treatment has stopped yet signs of tension occur at the time of boxing, offer the oils again. If the horse still turns away from them, other oils may be needed.

It may be helpful to have on hand a euphoric, calming blend: 3 drops of each of the following in 12ml of base oil – Jasmine, Frankincense, Vetiver and Violet Leaf.

Airborne bacteria

Warm, humid air inside the horsebox or trailer is a breeding ground for bacteria and a perfect environment for the transfer of disease. **Garlic** and **Bergamot** contain highly antiseptic molecules that help to provide a hostile environment for airborne bacteria and mites, thus deterring the spread of disease when travelling.

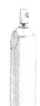

To help combat airborne bacteria, try the following recipe:

40 drops of Bergamot oil
10 drops Garlic oil
200ml water

Shake well. A disperser (supplied by essential oil specialists) can help to infuse the oil and water. When spraying into the air **avoid contact with the eyes.**

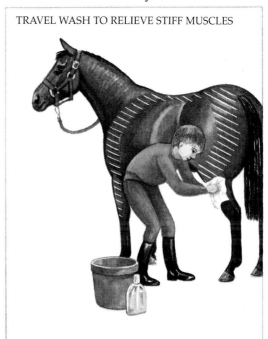

TRAVEL WASH TO RELIEVE STIFF MUSCLES

Birch – 20 drops (breaks down lactic acid)
Peppermint – 20 drops (stimulates circulation)
Juniper – 10 drops (reduces excess fluid)
Ginger – 5 drops (warming)

Muscles can be washed down using 30-40 drops of the above blend in a half a litre (1 pint) of warm water. Adding a dash of mild shampoo helps to disperse the oils.

Essential oil reference chart

Oil		Uses
BERGAMOT	☀ 💧	**O E** Balancing. Uplifting. Tumours. Warts. Sarcoids. **E** Helps to kill airborne bacteria.
CARROT SEED	💧	**O** Stimulates the healing process. Nourishes cells (useful for cell damage). Helps wounds that won't heal, and internal bleeding. **E** Apply externally in a base oil, to strengthen the hoof.
CHAMOMILE, GERMAN	💧	**E** Inflamed, irritated skin. Soothing. Anti-inflammatory. Open wounds.
CHAMOMILE, ROMAN	💧	**O E** Calming. Nervous stress that manifests in the skin or stomach. Horses that are prone to stress-related colic, flaky skin, bald patches. **E** Mud fever, sweet itch, etc.
CLARY SAGE	💧	**E** Nervous irritability. Nervous, panicky horses. (Violet Leaf is often a more effective first choice.)
EUCALYPTUS	💧	**E** Infections of the respiratory tract. Helps to destroy airborne bacteria. Opens up the airways. Useful for some allergy-related conditions especially when mixed with Great Mugwort.
FENNEL	△	**O** Digestive stimulant. Balances female function. Excessive or poor milk flow.
FRANKINCENSE	💧	**E** Past and present fears. Slows and deepens breathing. Calms coughs, especially if the breathing problem is due to anxiety.
GARLIC	△ 💧	**O** Immune stimulant. Worms. Blood thinner. **O E** Lung infection. **E** Kills airborne bacteria. Mites.
GRAPEFRUIT	☀ 💧	**O E** Refreshing, uplifting. **O** Internally cleansing. Associated with the liver. Helps to break down fats.
JASMINE	💧	**E** Helps to distance the mind from worries, fears and commotion. Horses that spend a lot of time stabled, or those that are prone to weaving, often respond to Jasmine.
JUNIPER BERRY	💧	**O** Excessive water intake and urination. Diuretic, so aids problems of fluid retention. Helps to clear toxins from the system. **E** Very effective, externally, for the treatment of arthritis and fluid retention.
LAVENDER	💧	**E** Soothing. Calming. Helps prevent scarring. Burns. Wounds. Skin disorders. Mild immune stimulant.
LEMON	☀ 💧	**O** Internally helps to break down kidney stones. Immune stimulant. Aids against winter chills. Cleansing. **E** Applied externally it is uplifting.
MUGWORT, GREAT	💧	**E** Rich dark blue in colour, do not use if clear. Natural anti-histamine therefore useful for the treatment of allergic conditions, COPD, laminitis, skin, etc.
NEROLI (Orange Blossom)	💧	**E** Sadness. Nervous disorders affecting the heart and/or stomach. Loss of companion. Loss of will to get better. Depression. Gives confidence.

NUTMEG	△	**O E** Influences dream activity. Together with Vetiver it helps to 'centre' horses with scattered energy. Also for horses that are bargy and difficult to hold back.
PATCHOULI	⊘	**O E** Viral or bacterial urinary infections. Warming and comforting.
PEPPERMINT	⊘	**E** Aches and sprains (do not use on open wounds). Anti-inflammatory, ice-pack/deep heat effect. Pain-killing properties. Stimulates nerve function. **O E** Stimulates circulation. Opens up respiratory airways; cleansing and stimulating to the lungs. Mental stimulant. **O** Digestive stimulant. Bowel disorders.
ROSE	⊘	**E** Resentment. Anger. Past trauma. Past abuse. Balances female function.
ROSEMARY	⊘	**O E** Stimulates circulation. Cleansing
SANDALWOOD	⊘	**E** Emotionally soothing and relaxing. Throat infections. **O** Strengthens bladder/kidneys. Its use may be indicated by excessive water intake and urination.
SEAWEED	💧	**O** Strong immune stimulant. Detoxifies. Nourishes the body with a cornucopia of nutrients and minerals. **O E** May be useful where there is poisoning.
TEA TREE	💧	**O E** Natural antibiotic. Antiseptic. Anti-viral. Anti-fungal. **E** Insect bites. Thrush. Ringworm. **O** Bladder/kidney infections, often indicated by excessive water intake and urination.
THYME	△ ⊘	**E** Strong antiseptic, only use when Tea Tree has been ineffective. May irritate healthy skin. Very effective in the treatment of severe lung infections. **O** Useful against some types of worms.
VETIVER	⊘	**E** Very grounding, deeply relaxing. Useful for the treatment of nervous tension.
VIOLET LEAF	⊘	**O E** Nervous, unsettled horses that spook easily. Horses that have been moved to a new home or yard. It comforts and strengthens the heart and is used for nervous exhaustion. A very popular oil with many horses. Its aroma resembles that of cut grass and cucumbers.
YARROW	💧	**E** Strong emotional release. Powerful anti-inflammatory and anti-bacterial properties, but gentle on the skin. Use on inflamed wounds, irritated skin and inflammation of tissue. Beneficial for itchy skin conditions and insect bites. A useful antidote for an adverse reaction to an essential oil. Urinary infections.
YLANG YLANG	⊘	**E** Comforting and relaxing. Distances worries, giving carefree feelings. Similar in its properties to Jasmine. Foals and yearlings will very often respond to Ylang Ylang, whereas older horses will more frequently respond to Jasmine.

All oils listed here may be licked off the hand if the horse chooses to do so (with the vet's approval). **Remember:** Always consult your vet before using essential oils.

KEY   **O** can be given orally   **E** apply externally   △ caution: possible skin irritant   💧 may be used undiluted

⊘ dilute well before use   ☀ caution: photosensitiser – avoid using on skin in strong sunlight; it may cause sunburn

Quick-reference selection charts

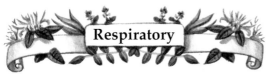

Respiratory

BERGAMOT : Cleansing. Airborne bacteria.
CARROT SEED : Cell damage, bleeding.
EUCALYPTUS : Infection. Fever. Some allergy-related conditions.
FRANKINCENSE : Calming to the lungs. Slows and deepens breathing.
GARLIC : Severe infection to the lungs. Airborne bacteria. Allergy-related conditions.
GREAT MUGWORT : Allergies. COPD. Anti-histamine.
PEPPERMINT : Cleansing. Stimulating. Opens up the airways. Allergy-related conditions.
TEA TREE : Anti-bacterial. Anti-fungal. Anti-viral.
THYME : Severe infection.

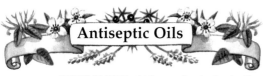

Antiseptic Oils

BERGAMOT : Airborne bacteria. Anti-bacterial.
EUCALYPTUS : Lung infection. Fever.
GARLIC : Infection. Airborne bacteria. Worms. Lungs.
JUNIPER : Kidney/urinary infection.
LEMON : Cleansing. Infections/winter chills.
SANDALWOOD : Throat/kidney/urinary infection.
TEA TREE : Natural antibiotic. Wounds. Fever. Fungal/viral infections. Insect bites. Urinary infection.
THYME : Lungs. Severe infection. Worms.
YARROW : Open pussy wounds. Urinary infection.

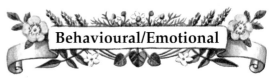

Behavioural/Emotional

BERGAMOT : Balancing. Uplifting.
CLARY SAGE : Nervousness. Panic.
FRANKINCENSE : Fear.
JASMINE : Deeply relaxing. Euphoric.
LAVENDER : Soothing.
NEROLI : Sadness. Loss of companion. Loss of will to recover.
NUTMEG : Euphoric. Scattered energy. Barging.
PEPPERMINT : Stimulating. Lethargy.
ROMAN CHAMOMILE : Stress/nervousness manifesting in the skin or stomach.
ROSE : Resentment. Anger. Past abuse. Past trauma. Mare-ish behaviour/irritability.
SANDALWOOD : Comforting. Relaxing.
VETIVER : Grounding.
VIOLET LEAF : Nervousness. Spooking. New home.
YARROW : Emotional release.
YLANG YLANG : Mainly used on colts. Deeply relaxing.

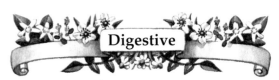

Digestive

FENNEL : Digestive stimulant.
FRANKINCENSE : Loose droppings.
GARLIC/THYME : Worms: severe infection.
NEROLI : Sadness. Stress-related colic.
PEPPERMINT : Digestive stimulant. Colon problems.
ROMAN CHAMOMILE : Nervous stomach. Colic.
SEAWEED : Poisoning. Detoxifier.
TEA TREE : Bacterial/viral infection.

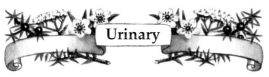

Urinary

CARROT SEED : Where there may be long-term damage.
JUNIPER : Diuretic. Detoxifier.
LEMON : Helps to break down stone-forming material. Antiseptic.
PATCHOULI : Vaginal/kidney/bladder infection.
SANDALWOOD : Structural/urinary infection.
TEA TREE : Natural antibiotic.
YARROW : Emotional/urinary infection. Anti-inflammatory.

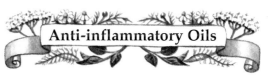

Anti-inflammatory Oils

PEPPERMINT : Eases inflammation by warming muscles and controlling blood flow. Aches/sprains/swelling. Pain-killing properties. Do **not** apply to **broken** skin.
GREAT MUGWORT : Anti-histamine. COPD. Laminitis. Skin conditions.
YARROW/GERMAN CHAMOMILE : Anti-inflammatory where tissues are swollen and injuries where skin is broken or unbroken. Pus-infected wounds. Sprains.

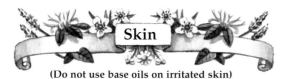

Skin

(Do not use base oils on irritated skin)

BERGAMOT : Tumours. Warts. Cysts. Sarcoids. Eczema.
CARROT SEED : Hoof strengthener (apply to hoof in base oil).
GARLIC : Mites. Midges. Use with German Chamomile or Yarrow to counteract the harsh effects of the Garlic on the skin.
GERMAN CHAMOMILE OR YARROW : Soothes broken, inflamed skin; helps dispel heat and ease pain. Very cleansing. Anti-bacterial.
GREAT MUGWORT : Anti-histamine; allergic reactions.
LAVENDER : Mites. Fleas. Proud flesh. Scarring. Mud fever. Sweet itch. Burns.
ROMAN CHAMOMILE : Stress-related skin disorders. Bald patches. Sweet itch. Mud fever. Stimulates hair growth.
TEA TREE : Mites. Insect bites. Dandruff. Ringworm. Thrush. Fungal infections. Mud fever. Sweet itch.

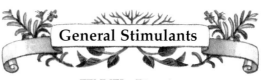

General Stimulants

FENNEL : Digestive.
PEPPERMINT : Central nervous system. Digestive. Blood.
ROSEMARY : Blood. Lymph.

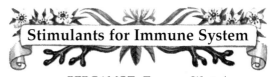

Stimulants for Immune System

BERGAMOT : Tumours.Warts/sarcoids.
CARROT SEED : Stimulates healing. Nourishes cells.
GARLIC : Powerful immune stimulant for infection.
LEMON : Run down. Winter chills.
SEAWEED : Detoxifier. Nourishes the body with a cornucopia of nutrients and minerals. Powerful immune stimulant.
TEA TREE : Natural antibiotic. Viral/fungal infections.

Quality and storage

It is very important to use top quality essential oils for optimum results. These do, however, have a price which often does not compete in the retail market. A label reading 'pure' or 'natural' is not necessarily a guard against poor quality oils which may have been adulterated with cheaper oils. Labels that read 'organic' or 'wild' are usually a wiser choice, as is a reputable supplier.

Essential oils oxidise, so lids should be firmly screwed on. The oils are in one sense 'living' and have a life span of approximately six months to five years depending on the oil and its quality. The lighter oils, especially citrus oils like Lemon, have the shortest life span, and the heavier oils, such as Sandalwood and Rose, have the longest. To determine if an oil has aged check for a slightly cloudy appearance which settles near the bottom of the bottle. Heavier oils should retain the full strength of the aroma.

Essential oils are also damaged by sunlight so should be bottled in opaque (dark) bottles or glass that contains UV protection. They should be kept in a cool, dark place. This will help to ensure a longer shelf-life.

Those interested in finding out more about equine aromatherapy can contact the Equine Aromatherapy Association, PO Box 19, Hay-on-Wye, Hereford, HR3 5AE, UK.

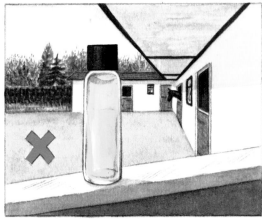

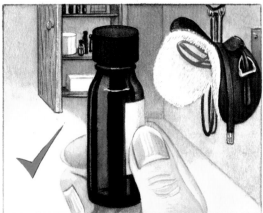

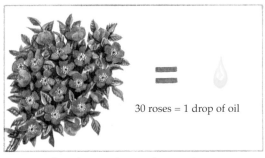

30 roses = 1 drop of oil

30 Rose heads = 1 drop of Rose Otto essential oil (clear in colour). Rose Otto is expensive to make, therefore a cheap oil must be questioned. Rose absolute (orange in colour) is extracted by a different method which gives a higher yield. This oil is not as pure, but is still of therapeutic value.